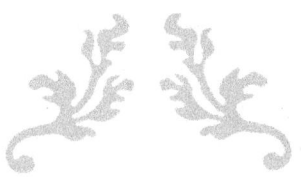

INTERMITTENT FASTING

The Complete Guide for Beginners to
Weight Loss and Healthy Eating Mastery

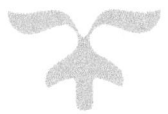

WRITTEN BY
Dr. Jason Sanders

Table of Contents

Introduction

Do you want to give intermittent fasting (IF) a try? Then you will be delighted to know that it has a lot of rewarding benefits, especially in your overall fitness and physique. In fact, a huge increase in the number of its proponents says that IF helped them accelerate fat loss while also improving their overall health.

Aside from helping you achieve your target weight, IF also contributes to increasing your energy and enjoying several health benefits. Add to that the fact that this eating pattern is not expensive and does not consume a lot of your time. If you are genuinely interested to try out this famous health and fitness trend then consider gathering lots of relevant information about it first so you will know if it is suitable for you.

Luckily, you can now gather as much information as you want about IF through this e-book, *"Intermittent Fasting: An Essential Guide for Beginners"*. Through this book, you will know exactly what IF is, how it functions, the benefits it can give, and the different IF methods that you can try. It even tackles its short history, giving you a background of when and how it actually started.

By reading this book, you can collect tips on how to start your journey towards better health and fitness through IF. Furthermore, you will know whether it is indeed the appropriate fitness program for you. It will also tackle any side effects of IF and how to deal with them.

Overall, this book will serve as a comprehensive guide that will make sticking to this lifestyle more manageable. You will be guided on what to do so you can maximize the results of IF.

Chapter 1 – A Brief History of Intermittent Fasting

Before we go over the details of intermittent fasting (how it works, how to begin doing it, its benefits, etc.), it helps to try learning a bit about its history so you will have some background on when it started and why it became popular. Fasting is actually an old concept already. In fact, several forms of fasting were already practiced by various religious groups in different parts of the world for centuries.

A lot of medical practitioners also noted the advantages of fasting for hundreds and thousands of year. This means that fasting for fitness can't be considered as a new fad in dieting or an ineffective marketing ploy. Humans fasted for the majority of their history whether it is for religious purposes, just a typical overnight fasting period, or an extended period due to food scarcity.

What is new is that there are now some clinical studies showing the benefits of intermittent fasting for a person's longevity, fitness, and overall health. It has been reported that when properly done, intermittent fasting can't only lead to losing weight or managing your body weight but also in extending your life, regulating blood glucose, maintaining or gaining lean mass, and controlling blood lipids, among other rewarding health benefits.

Intermittent fasting also started to gain popularity in the United Kingdom in 2012 after the Eat, Fast, and Live Longer documentary was broadcasted on BBC2 television. It also became a trend in the US, particularly in Silicon Valley Companies. As of the moment, the interest in IF continues to rise, causing companies to commercialize dietary supplements, full meal packages, and diet coaching that is compatible with IF.

One more thing to take note of about intermittent fasting for fitness and weight loss is that it originated from the belief that it does not only support weight loss but also provides your body with enough time to detoxify from what you have eaten and practiced the night before. It is because of its ability to clear your body from waste products, like carbon dioxide, lactic acid, and toxins from junk and unhealthy foods.

It clears your blood vessels, allowing protein as well as other essential vitamins and nutrients to flow smoothly and easily through your body. With the benefits discovered from practicing intermittent fasting, it is no longer surprising why it became popular, leading to the development of its different variations that further maximize its positive effects.

Chapter 2 – What is Intermittent Fasting and How Does it Work?

One thing that you should know about intermittent fasting is that you can't consider it as a diet plan. In fact, it is an eating pattern, which requires you to schedule your meals to maximize their positive effects on your fitness and health. The pattern involves a cycle composed of separate periods of eating and fasting. So basically, this eating pattern does not require you to change the foods you eat. What you need to change is actually your eating schedule.

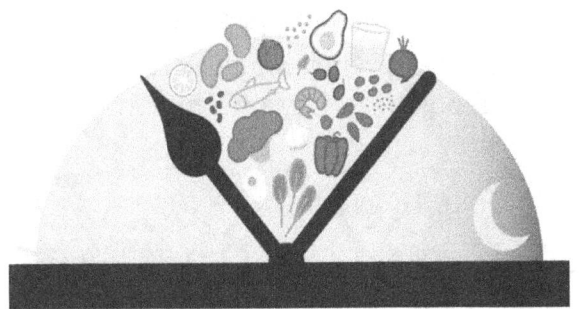

Now, you may be asking yourself if it is really worthwhile to make some changes on when you should eat. The answer is actually a resounding yes. In fact, IF is an incredible solution if you want to be lean and stay that way without having to follow crazy and difficult diet plans or focus too much on counting calories. In most cases, this eating pattern even requires you to retain your calorie intake when you are still starting out.

In addition, it is a great way of preserving your muscle mass while still keeping your body lean. It is also the simplest strategy if you want to take off unwanted weight and ensure that you stay within your target. You can do that without making excessive changes in your behavior. This makes intermittent fasting simple and doable in the sense that anyone can easily do it while still remaining meaningful as it truly creates a positive difference in your weight and health.

How Does IF Work?

Learning about the fasted and the fed state is the key to recognizing the way IF works specifically and how it results in weight loss. Note that your body is in its fed state each time it is in the process of food absorption and digestion. It begins when you start to eat. It tends to last for around 3-5 hours while your body works on digesting and absorbing all the foods you consumed. Note that during the fed state, your body will have a difficult time burning fat because of your high insulin level.

After completing the fed state, your body will be in the post-absorptive state. It refers to the time when your body does not process a meal. This state lasts for around 8-12 hours after you have taken your last meal. This is also the time when you get into the fasted state.

Your body will have an easier time burning fat during the fasted state since it is also the time when you have low insulin levels. It is even the time when your body can stimulate the process of burning those fats that were inaccessible while you are still in your fed state.

Since you can't get into the fasted state until twelve hours have passed since your last meal, it would be a rare case for your body to be in a fat burning state. With this notion, it is no longer surprising why those who begin IF lose fat even if they did not change how much and what they eat and the frequency and duration of their exercises. Through fasting, it is possible for your body to get into the fat burning state, which you can't usually achieve when you are following your normal eating schedule.

Chapter 3 – Benefits of Intermittent Fasting

Intermittent fasting can shower you with plenty of pleasant and rewarding benefits. It allows you to have full control of your health while letting you more mindful about your eating patterns and when you should eat. What is even greater about intermittent fasting is that it was the eating pattern adopted by our ancestors, which just proves that it works and it allows you to survive.

It lets you embrace famine and feast cycles so you can work in a preventive manner as a means of resetting the hormones needed for better metabolism. This also allows your body to have a break from digesting foods. Regularly adopting intermittent fasting can even provide you with numerous physical and mental benefits.

To learn more specifically about what it can do, this chapter will cover some of the benefits that you can enjoy from sticking to IF.

Supports your Weight Loss Journey

Of course, one of the most prominent benefits of intermittent fasting is that it drives weight loss. It does so by keeping your insulin level low. Note that your body tends to break down carbs into glucose that your body cells utilize to produce energy or convert them into fat with the aim of storing it for later use. Insulin refers to a hormone, which lets your cells absorb glucose.

If you do not consume or eat food then it is greatly possible for your insulin level to drop. This increases the possibility of the reduced insulin level to trigger the release of glucose stores in the form of energy during the fasting period. If this process happens on a regular basis, just like when you are doing IF, then it will eventually result in significant weight loss.

You can also expect intermittent fasting to support your weight loss journey because it can encourage you to consume fewer calories. It is because you will also be eating fewer meals. Furthermore, this eating pattern can improve the way your hormones function, thereby facilitating weight loss. Short-term fasting can even lead to an increase in your metabolic rate, giving you the chance to burn a higher amount of calories.

Good for your Mental Health

Another incredible benefit of intermittent fasting is that it can improve your brain function and mental health. Keep in mind that as you age, your brain will also receive less blood flow. The aging process can result in the shrinking of neurons and the decline in your brain volume. Through IF, it is possible to delay the aging process, which is useful in sharpening your brain and keeping your mental health at an all-time high.

Because of its positive effects on your brain and mental health, this eating pattern can also contribute to lowering your risk of suffering from neurodegenerative diseases, like Parkinson's and Alzheimer's disease. It is because it can also prevent obesity and diabetes – both of which are among the factors that can trigger the development of neurodegenerative diseases.

Practicing IF can also prevent nerve cell degeneration, thereby keeping your brain as healthy as possible. It can improve your memory and your ability to learn. This eating pattern also contributes to improving your mood, thereby lowering your risk of suffering from depression. Furthermore, it can boost your mental alertness and give you some sense of peace especially during the fasting period.

Promotes Longevity

Another positive effect of intermittent fasting is that it allows you to live a longer life. It is because it can protect you from different kinds of ailments – among which are heart diseases, diabetes, and cancer. One thing that it can do for your health that will eventually lengthen your life is lowering your bad cholesterol level. It also lowers your blood pressure and insulin resistance.

Together with chemotherapy, it is also possible for IF to slow down skin and breast cancer progression. It is because it raises the number of tumor-infiltrating lymphocytes in your body that refer to cells that your immune system sends as a means of attacking the tumor that causes cancer.

IF also works in making your cells resilient, thereby delaying the aging process and increasing your lifespan along the process. It allows your body to process energy in a more efficient manner, which leads to vibrant aging and longevity.

Simplifies your Life

Another reason why intermittent fasting is worthwhile to try is that it works in simplifying your life. It can lessen your stress level as there are times within the day, especially the fasting hours when you no longer have to think about what to cook or where to grab food.

For instance, if your fasting period is breakfast then your mornings will be less complicated since you no longer have to worry about what to eat once you wake up. You can already start your day with just a glass of water. Taking even just a single meal out of your worries can already save a significant amount of your time and can simplify your life.

Develops a More Structured Eating Pattern

Do you often find yourself snacking in between meals mindlessly? It could be the slice of cake that goes with your regular coffee, some dried fruits and nuts prior to eating your dinner, or some popcorn during a movie night. If you really think it through, those little snacks that you take in mindlessly might actually increase your calorie intake.

Fortunately, you can now try intermittent fasting, which allows you to eat in a more structured manner. With this, you can eliminate the problem linked to mindless eating and increased calorie intake, thereby giving you full control of your diet.

Guarantees More Satisfying Meals

Through intermittent fasting, you no longer have to eat every two to three hours, which is actually inconvenient and impractical for many, especially those who have extremely busy schedules. You can also stop yourself from eating huge meals too frequently even if you are physically inactive.

Intermittent fasting can lead to larger volumes of meals because you will be making up for the long periods of fasting. These bigger meals are actually more satisfying and capable of making you feel fuller for quite a longer period.

Improves Hunger Awareness

If you take frequent meals all throughout the day then there is a high chance for you to eat for other reasons apart from hunger. For instance, you might be eating just because you are stressed, sad, or bored. You may also eat because you are happy.

With intermittent fasting, you will be more aware of your own body cues that signal hunger. You will know exactly what it feels like to experience real hunger. It also gives you the chance to differentiate real hunger from simple cravings brought on by psychological and environmental factors.

Apart from the indicated benefits, IF can also have a significant impact on your life by encouraging cellular repair, reducing inflammation and oxidative stress, preventing Type 2 diabetes, and improving your cardiovascular function. Now that you are completely aware of its positive effects, it is the perfect time to move on to learning its different kinds so you will know which one suits you the most.

Chapter 4 – Different Types of Intermittent Fasting

Intermittent fasting boasts of several well-known benefits including the ones mentioned in the previous chapter. It helps lose stubborn fats, curb cravings, lower inflammation, and improve gut micro-biome. It involves abstaining from foods for certain periods. While it is tough to do at first, you will get used to it eventually, especially if you choose to practice the most suitable type of IF for you.

This chapter will cover the most popular types or methods of intermittent fasting and an overview of each one so you can figure out which one is tailored perfectly to suit your unique personality and lifestyle.

16/8 Method

One of the most widely practiced types of intermittent fasting is the 16/8 method. Otherwise referred to as the Leangains method, the 16/8 requires you to fast for 16 hours every day and eat your meals within an 8-hour window. Some do this approach by skipping breakfast then restricting their daily food consumption within an 8-hour period. This allows them to fast for up to 16 hours.

It should be noted that how you schedule your fasting period and eating window is up to you. If you consider dinner as a vital part of your daily routine then you may skip your breakfast. However, if you are someone who tends to get cranky if you do not eat a healthy breakfast then it would be ideal to skip dinner instead.

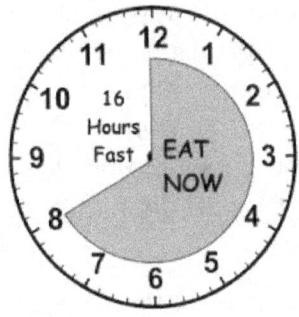

The majority of those who followed the 16/8 approach, though, noticed that it is much more convenient and easier if they prolong their fasting schedule during the morning and eat their first meal at lunch.

In fact, over 2/3 of those who follow the famous 16/8 intermittent fasting method prefer to skip breakfast and eat meals only around lunch.

One thing to remember, though, is that you do not have to be extremely strict when trying to follow this approach. In fact, you are allowed to make some slight changes in the fasting and feeding periods. For instance, you may choose to fast for just 14 hours and have an eating window of 10 hours.

Note that the premise of this approach is to simply lessen the time spent on eating and fast for most times of the day. You can repeat this IF method as frequently as possible. You can even choose to do it just once or two times every week depending on your personal preference.

Another thing to remember is that it might take several days for you to find out the right fasting and eating windows that work for you, especially if you are someone who leads an extremely active lifestyle or if you tend to get hungry once you wake up in the morning.

protein, veggies, and healthy fats to avoid any carb cravings or a significant drop in your blood sugar level.

Also, do not fast during those days when you are planning to do plenty of endurance exercises. In case you are planning to run a race or bike on a particularly day, find out first if this fasting method is compatible with your workout plan before starting. You can also talk to your sports nutritionist about it just to be safe.

Alternate Day Fasting

As its name suggests, alternate day fasting involves fasting for the entire day then following your normal eating habits the next day. In other words, the first day should involve consuming water and a total of 500 calories with 200 of such intake taken from protein sources. You can take this 500-calorie requirement in just a single meal or spread it out the entire day.

On the second day, you can eat normally again. It is advisable to stick to this routine every two days. But come to think of it, there are a couple of ways to implement this approach. The first one is completely fasting during the fasting day. This means you should only drink water during this period.

Another approach is to eat small meals (a max of 25 percent compared to your regular intake of calories). On average, this is roughly 500 to 600 calories. Just make sure that you do not include starches or sugar in the 25 percent limit.

24-hour Fasting

Clearly, this fasting method requires you to fast for 24 hours, meaning it lasts from breakfast to breakfast or dinner to dinner depending on your preference. For instance, you will eat a healthy breakfast at around 8 am and fast until 8 am the next day. This approach does not actually mean that you will go on the entire day without eating. It is because you still eat a full meal within that fasting day.

There are several advantages to the 24-hour fasting. The first one is that it is more effective compared to the others because the fasting duration is longer. You still eat daily, although it will just be one full meal at a consistent schedule. Since you are still eating, you can take the medications that need to go along with meals. For instance, if you need to take aspirin or iron supplements, then you can take them together with that one full meal.

You can also easily incorporate this IF approach into your daily lifestyle. For instance, if you decide to eat your one full meal at dinner then you just fast routinely for 24 hours hassle-free and without anyone noticing the difference in your lifestyle. It is because you just need to skip breakfast and lunch that day. The approach is often perfect during workdays. You can just drink your coffee or tea then skip breakfast.

You can then do what you needed to do at work until you reach home to eat your dinner with family. It is a convenient approach while also allowing you to save a lot of time, money, and effort. You no longer need to clean up or cook for a couple of meals a day. It is also possible for you to save some time during lunchtime that you can just dedicate to work. Without anyone noticing that you actually fasted for a max of 24 hours, you can finally reach home and enjoy your full dinner.

If you want to use this approach to lose weight then it is advisable to do this fasting approach at least three times weekly. Some of those who follow this approach even choose to do it 5 times weekly or even daily. In your case, you have to figure out what fits your schedule the most and your weight loss goals.

The Warrior Diet

The warrior diet refers to an IF protocol, which comes with extended fasting periods and short feasting periods. During the feast, it is advisable to consume around 85-90 percent of your required calorie consumption. This can reach 1,800 calories in a single sitting if you are following the standard 2,000-calorie meal plan.

The calorie intake may also go up to 2,700 calories if you are extremely active, making it necessary for you to consume up to 3,000 calories daily. Many view the warrior diet as a more rigid form of IF since it alternates 20 hours of under-eating and four hours of unlimited food consumption. In most cases, the fasting period happens at night and the entire day. The 4-hour feasting period usually happens during the evening.

It follows the concept of our ancestors who spent a lot of time during the day hunting for food then eating what they gathered at night. The problem is because of the long fasting period, which causes you to under-eat, and the unlimited food consumption during the feasting period, nutrient deficiencies might occur. This is the main reason why the warrior diet does not suit some groups of people, such as pregnant women and athletes.

With the risk of nutrient-deficiency, it is advisable to focus on eating foods rich in nutrients. You can do so by sticking to protein sources as well as fruits and veggies. Your daily meals should also include healthy fats and dairy sources of protein, like yogurt and cheese. The good thing about the warrior diet is that it does not require you to count calories provided you stick to the recommended foods to be included in your meals and avoid unprocessed foods.

Prolonged Fasting

Prolonged fasting is also a popular approach among those who are into intermittent fasting - with one in every four of them implementing this approach. As its name suggests, it involves longer periods of fasting. It involves at least 24 hours without food intake.

You can even try the 36-hour fast, which is also a popular version of prolonged fasting. This involves fasting for a total of 36 hours. For instance, your last meal on the first day is at 8 pm. You will have to skip all meals on the second day. You will only eat on the third day at exactly 8 am, completing the 36-hour fasting period.

What is good about this longer period of fasting is that it offers quick results, especially in weight loss. It is also ideal for Type 2 diabetics who are known for having more resistance to insulin.

You can also try the 42-hour fasting period and beyond. There are those who were able to carry out fasting for longer periods (up to 42 hours and sometimes more). It especially happens for those who tried the

16/8 pattern who noticed after several days of sticking to the program that they feel normal even after they just begin their daily routines with water and coffee.

Combining that with the 36-hour fasting routine will cause you to fast for a total of 42 hours. For instance, your dinner on the first day, which also served as your last meal during your eating period, is at 7 pm. On the second day, you will need to skip all your meals. You should only eat your next meal at 1 pm. You can also go for a fasting duration, which is longer than the 42 hours but it is advisable to avoid restricting your calorie intake during your next eating period.

Note that while you get used to the fasting pattern, your appetite may also go down. With that in mind, it is advisable to eat to your contentment during the eating day. The decrease in your appetite is because of the reduced level of insulin during the time when your insulin resistance cycle is broken down due to fasting. Note that insulin plays a major role in regulating your body weight, so it is no longer surprising for your body to go lower now.

This results to a suppression in hunger and the maintenance in your total energy expenditure. Note that you have the option to extend your fast for a longer period, depending on what you can handle comfortably. There are even those who are capable of fasting for 7-14 days without any problem. Just make sure that the longer fasting period suits your lifestyle and present health condition before trying it out. If possible, consult your doctor first so you can figure out its suitability to your condition.

Chapter 5 – Who Should Try Intermittent Fasting?

Intermittent fasting is indeed one of the best ways to achieve your target weight but you can't expect it to work for everyone. For example, it may not suit those who are pregnant or have serious health conditions that might worsen with continued fasting. Generally, the IF pattern works best for those who are generally fit and want to maintain their current weight.

It also works for those whose body figures are on the overweight and obese side as they are the ones who wish to shed off some pounds through fasting. It does not work for those who are already underweight, so find out whether your current weight is suitable for IF before starting it out.

Provided your current body and health condition are suitable for IF, you will notice that it is a great way to gain insights on distinguishing simple cravings and real hunger. This will prevent you from having to give in to your unhealthy cravings since you are already aware of when you are really hungry.

Another thing you have to remember about intermittent fasting is that it will most likely lead to success if you are someone who already experienced monitoring your food and calorie intake in the past. It is appropriate for experienced exercisers or those whose present jobs allow low-performance periods. It is also perfect for you if you are single and do not have kids yet. These scenarios and personalities can lead to a successful intermittent fasting journey since these will let you adapt the pattern easily.

You can also try intermittent fasting even if you already have kids or are married, an athlete or a sports enthusiast, or someone whose job requires you to deliver an excellent performance most of the time. However, you have to apply the pattern with caution. It is because your present situation might pose some challenges in sticking to the pattern.

If you are into sports then your performance may also be affected during the fasting period. Women should also be extra cautious when doing intermittent fasting as this might cause them to experience unwanted side effects, like hormonal imbalance, irregular periods, anxiety, and sleeplessness. If you are a female interested in IF then it is advisable to start this approach in a relaxed manner to avoid the mentioned negative effects.

Who Should Avoid IF?

While there are a lot of people who continue to enjoy a lot of benefits from intermittent fasting, there are also those who should avoid it at all costs. If your body type is on the underweight side then do not bother trying IF as this might only have a negative impact on your weight and overall health. It is also advisable to try other eating patterns or dieting approaches, instead of IF, in case you are:

- **Pregnant** – Note that your pregnancy requires you to supply your body with more than enough energy and nutrition so it is not advisable to fast during this period.

- **Experienced disordered eating in the past** – If you experienced eating disorders in the past, then you should avoid thinking about fasting. Keep in mind that a fasting protocol might only trigger more issues in your eating pattern in the future. It might even mess up your health, so it would be best to look for other ways to manage your weight.

- **Someone whose new into exercising and dieting** – If you are still a beginner in both exercising and dieting, then IF might appear like the best weight loss solution for you. However, it would be best to find out how to deal with nutritional deficiencies prior to experimenting with IF. You need to have a solid and reliable nutritional platform first before you begin to fast.

Aside from the ones mentioned, the following are also among those who should abstain from IF:

- Those who are chronically stressed and experience problems getting adequate sleep

- Breastfeeding moms

- People who need to take medications with proper meals

- Adolescents or those who are in the active growth phase

- Those who have endocrinological issues

- Cardiac disease or congestive heart failure patients

To find out if intermittent fasting is a safe eating pattern for you, try to consult a nutritionist or your doctor before starting the routine. You have to get a go-signal first to ensure that your health and body will not be compromised.

Chapter 6 – How to Maximize the Benefits of Intermittent Fasting?

Once you have consulted a certified nutritionist or your doctor and you gained their approval for trying intermittent fasting then you have to arm yourself with the right knowledge about how it works so you can use it to your best advantage. So how can you really maximize the benefits of intermittent fasting? Adapt it while keeping in mind these tips:

Start small and in a slow and simple manner

Intermittent fasting takes a lot of discipline and getting used to, so you should avoid rushing into the process. Start small and do it on a simple and gradual manner. Choose to do one small and simple thing related to IF to begin with. For instance, you can start by making adjustments on your regular meal schedules by 1-2 hours. There is no need to do a drastic change right away. Find out if the adjustment works and slowly work towards following your preferred IF method.

You also need to get to know more about yourself first. Spend time carefully observing your own experiences. Prior to starting, it is necessary to gather as much data and insights as possible. The information you gathered will help you in drawing conclusions that you will find useful in executing your future action once you start the IF approach. Just remember to take your time. In fact, some spent several weeks before they finally mastered the new program and made it a part of their lifestyle.

Determine the results you want to achieve

Avoid starting intermittent fasting if you do not have a clear idea about the results you wish to achieve. Know exactly what you want to gain from practicing IF. By knowing your preferred outcome, you get the chance to pick the most suitable IF method for you.

You can try intermittent fasting if you wish to delve deeper into the physical and psychological experiences associated with hunger. Intermittent fasting is also the right approach if you wish to attain the following results:

- Learn to distinguish between actual hunger and simple cravings

- Let go of your fear of hunger

- Improve sensitivity to insulin

- Recalibrate the use of stored fuel within your body

- Understand the eating process and respect the privilege of being able to do so

- Gain a deeper understanding about your body

- Achieve your target weight

- Free yourself from the hassle of food preparation

Know exactly what your objectives are before starting IF as it will also help you create a plan that will lead you to your preferred results. However, you also have to take note that no matter how good your goals are, you can't expect intermittent fasting to work effectively and safely in achieving them if you are also doing the following:

- Using "health" as an excuse for your eating disorder or for strictly controlling your food intake

- Fasting too often for extremely long periods of time

- Exercising excessively or having insufficient sleep

- Over-obsessing with food or binging once your feeding or eating period arrives

- Taking appetite suppressants to avoid extreme difficulty during the fasting period

- Using intermittent fasting as an excuse for overeating or unhealthy and poor food choices and eating patterns

You have to set healthy goals for adapting intermittent fasting. Avoid doing it to compromise your health. The first thing to do is to set a healthy goal then learn the basics of nutrition. Make sure to consume healthy and high-quality foods at the right time and amounts.

Choose the right foods

During your eating period, it is important to eat the right foods. Make each calorie that your body takes in count. In case you choose an IF pattern, which gives you the chance to take in calories during the fasting state, then go for nutrient-dense foods, particularly those with high amounts of healthy fats, fiber, and protein. Some examples are eggs, avocado, nuts, fish, beans, and lentils.

You should also pick nutrient-dense foods rich in fiber, minerals, vitamins, and other essential nutrients that can stabilize your blood sugar during the eating period. The foods should help prevent nutritional deficiency. It is also advisable to pick filling foods with low calorie content, like raw vegetables and popcorn. You can also include fruits that have high water content, like melon and grapes in your meals.

To enjoy the fed state, make sure to improve the taste of the foods you are planning to eat without necessarily increasing their calorie content. You can do that by generously seasoning your meals with herbs, vinegar, spices, and garlic. This will allow your foods to be filled with flavor without increasing calories. It also helps in reducing your hunger.

Ensure that you stay hydrated, too. Drink enough water and low-calorie drinks, like herbal teas all throughout the day.

Do not pressure yourself to perfect the eating pattern

Avoid freaking out and pressuring yourself to perfect everything, especially if you are still a beginner in IF. If you intend to follow the 16/8 rule, for instance, then do not freak out in case you were just able to fast for 14 to 15 hours on a particular day. Do not also bombard yourself with unnecessary questions, like whether or not the result will be ruined in case you ate one apple during your fasting period.

To make the whole eating pattern more manageable, try to relax. Keep in mind that the human body is a machinery that learns to adapt as time goes by. You cannot expect it to follow the routine right away, especially if you are still new to it. Do not force yourself to stick to really rigid fasting rules. For instance, if you wish to enjoy eating your breakfast one day and fast on another, then allow yourself to do it.

Note that while you need to be more disciplined, especially if you really want to lose weight, you should avoid freaking out and worrying and stressing over every minute detail of the process. Just relax and you will notice your body starting to adapt to the new routine and the IF working in your favor slowly but surely.

Listen to your body

If you intend to stick to intermittent fasting for quite a long period then make it a point to listen and observe the cues sent to you by your body. Some of the cues you have to watch out for are significant changes in your satiety, hunger, and appetite, such as food cravings, your emotional or mental health and mood, the quality of your sleep, your athletic performance, and your energy levels. Make it a point to observe your immunity, hormonal health, blood profile, and the way you look, too.

Observing and listening to your body can help you figure out whether IF is working for you. If you are into strength training, then you have to listen to body cues even more. Find out if you experience lightheadedness during your workout. If that happens, it would be helpful to consume enough water.

Also, act right away if there is a noticeable drop in your performance. If that is the case, make it a point to consume enough calories, particularly those coming from protein and healthy fats during your eating window. Stop working out if your body feels extremely off. Allow yourself to have time to ease and get used to fasted workouts and IF. This tip is even more important, especially for endurance athletes.

Avoid overdoing your workouts

Just like what we have talked about in the previous tips, it is necessary to listen to the signals sent by your body. This is all the more necessary if you decide to combine your workout with fasting. Note that intermittent fasting and regular workout combined can produce better and quicker weight loss results. However, you should avoid overdoing your workouts, so you will not end up harming your body.

If you wish to work out and pair it with IF, then make sure to take into consideration all the things that are happening in your life. Consider the specific amount and intensity of training and exercise you do. Consider your rest and recovery period, too. You should also take into consideration the suitability of intermittent fasting with your normal social activities and regular routines as well as the other stress and demands that life throws at you. By considering all these factors, you can figure out what type of workout is compatible with your lifestyle and your preferred IF method.

Do not deprive yourself

Your decision to practice intermittent fasting does not necessarily mean that you should deprive yourself with even a drink during your fasted period. Note that it is okay to drink water and zero-calorie beverages. You can drink black coffee, tea, or water when you are fasting. Do not also stop yourself from putting something in your drink (like milk in your coffee).

Furthermore, remember that you are also allowed to drink diet soda on an occasional basis when you are fasting. Note that the goal here is habit-building and consistency. This means that if you feel like you can go through the fasting period more easily with a cream or milk in your coffee then there is no reason to deprive yourself.

Also, remember that adhering to the routine 80 percent of the time for a whole year is actually better than adhering to it 100 percent but only abandoning it after just a few weeks due to it being too rigid and restrictive. You can be stricter if you intend to reach a minimum percentage of body fat. However, if you want to achieve your goal at your own pace then do the things that you think will make you remain compliant to it for a long time.

Eat filling and satiating meals

Your meals can greatly affect your ability to stick to your fasting and dieting routines.

This is the main reason why you have to make sure that the meals and foods you eat during the eating window are all filling and satiating. Among the foods that can satisfy and fill you up during your eating window are eggs, yogurt, potatoes, oatmeal, bananas and soups.

You may also eat those foods that you can consume in large amounts without taking in a lot of calories, including legumes, fruits and veggies. This does not mean, however, that you should go all out when it comes to eating. You should still try limiting yourself without over-deprivation. This will allow you to enjoy your experience when following your chosen intermittent fasting method, thereby allowing you to stick to it for quite a long period.

Keep yourself busy

Your boredom will be your number one enemy when you are doing intermittent fasting that's why you have to do something to keep yourself busy during your fasting period. Boredom is also the silent killer, which might destroy your progress gradually. It might cause you to eat more than what is recommended without even realizing it. It is mainly because of dopamine, one of the chemicals in your brain, which can make you feel good each time you accomplish something. This chemical is also responsible for the behavior motivated by reward.

It has been discovered that eating is actually a major factor in encouraging your body to release dopamine, producing the positive feelings as a result. In most cases, unhealthy and junk foods, especially those rich in sodium, fat, and sugar, are the ones that can make you feel great. Therefore, if you are bored during your fasting period then there is a great possibility that you will grab a food no matter how hard you resist the temptation.

With that in mind, make sure that you are busy with something during the fasting period. Do not just sit around and think about your hunger since you may only struggle in the end. It would also be best to time your fasting period in a way that you can maximize its efficiency and minimize discomfort. For instance, schedule it after you have eaten a nice dinner so you have more time to fast without having to think about food since it is already close to your bedtime.

Develop an exit strategy

If you wish to follow intermittent fasting for a long time, then make sure to develop a plan that will guide and help you in reintroducing a regular eating schedule into your daily routines. Avoid committing the mistakes of those who fasted in the past who tend to trip up after deciding to break free from the IF cycle since they have a hard time reacquainting with their own hunger signals and appetite.

With that in mind, it would be a big help to develop an exit plan once you are done with intermittent fasting, especially if you prefer to do it the mindful and healthy way. You should also keep track of your progress and the results of practicing IF, too, so you will know exactly when the right time to stop is.

Intermittent fasting is indeed an incredible eating pattern, especially for those who wish to lose weight. The problem is that while others can easily do the fast without trouble and without experiencing too many irresistible food temptations, there are also those who find the whole process difficult. If you feel like you need a bit of help to succeed then you can always apply the tips mentioned in this chapter.

That way, you have a better chance of keeping your hunger at bay, preventing mindless eating even if you are hungry, gaining full control of your nutrition, and sticking to the routine, thereby allowing you to enjoy and maximize its results.

Chapter 7 - Intermittent Fasting Myths

Intermittent fasting is one of the most rewarding eating patterns and lifestyle you can try. However, before starting your journey towards enjoying its numerous benefits, it is crucial to study the facts and myths behind it. This chapter will debunk some of the most famous intermittent fasting myths and offer truthful information about how this eating pattern really works.

Myth #1 – Intermittent fasting guarantees significant weight loss.

Contrary to what most people believe, IF can't be expected to result in significant weight loss all the time. This is especially true if you are doing this approach the wrong way. Note that regardless of the length of your fast, you can't still expect to achieve the results you want as far as weight loss is concerned if you constantly include burgers, candies, pizzas, and other unhealthy foods during your eating period. You still need to pair IF with regular exercises and a healthy diet. You can't treat each eating period as a cheat day.

Myth #2 – Intermittent fasting leads to muscle loss.

No, your muscles will not shrivel up and break down during your fasted state. Keep in mind that the human body stores two forms of energy, namely fat and sugar. This means that your body will only be using these two forms of stored energy.

Protein, which is a major component of your muscles, will not be used by your body to produce energy when you are fasting. What happens, instead, is that your body will make use of sugar as the primary source of fuel during the first 1-2 days without food.

After that, your body will begin opening up and accessing stored fats as a source of energy. This means that it will start breaking down the stored fats in your body to create fuel once your stored sugar depletes. Each person has around 50,000 to 100,000 calories of fat on average stored in his body, which is equal to almost one month's worth of available stored fats.

If you intend to fast, therefore, then you do not have to worry about your muscles breaking down since it is your stored fat and sugar that your body will use as fuel.

Myth #3 – Intermittent fasting can slow down your metabolism.

You do not have to worry about intermittent fasting negatively affecting your metabolic rate. It is because the entire eating pattern will not slow down your metabolism. Keep in mind that IF does not involve excessive calorie restrictions. What it does is to restrict the time you consume calories.

A few more hours spent waiting to take your first meal does not have a major effect on your metabolic rate. However, you should avoid under-eating during your eating period as this practice is the one that might send your metabolism downhill.

Myth #4 – Intermittent fasting can lead to poor brain performance.

Glucose is your brain's main source of fuel. With that in mind, it is no longer surprising to see those who are planning to try IF worrying about being unable to give their brain a consistent supply of glucose. The truth, however, is that IF will not negatively affect the performance of your brain.

Keep in mind that your body is still capable of using stored fuel from your body to produce glucose. This means that even if you follow low-carb intermittent fasting approach, it is still possible for your brain to get a good supply of fuel through ketone bodies that break down fat.

Intermittent fasting can even lead to better mental performance, focus, and clarity. It is mainly because fasting can stimulate epinephrine and norepinephrine production. If you get into the fasting mode, your body will cause a minor stress response, which releases adrenaline. This breaks down the fats stored in your body as fuel, thereby providing you with the focus and energy you need.

Furthermore, fasting can lead to the production of BDNF (brain-derived neurotropic factor). This can help your existing neurons survive, stimulate the growth of new neurons, and improve your learning and thinking ability and your memory. It also helps lessen your risk of suffering from depression and Alzheimer's disease.

Myth #5 – You have limitless options during your eating window.

Some of those who tried intermittent fasting wrongly believed that they are allowed to eat whatever they want provided they consume it during the eating window. This is actually not true. In fact, eating without limitations during the eating window can only have serious consequences to your health, wellness, and weight loss goals. Eating anything during the eating period might cause your body to get confused.

It is because from being on a fasting state that results in balanced levels of blood glucose and fat burning, your body suddenly experiences a spike in insulin and blood glucose. If this happens, you are just basically ruining the incredible effort you have exerted for fasting.

Furthermore, not controlling the amount of food you eat during your eating window can make you feel terrible and produce issues, like weight gain, mood swings, and hormonal imbalance. Note that while intermittent fasting does not require you to be extremely strict during your eating window, you still have to balance the foods you eat. It is still crucial to apply moderation as this can help you gather the results you want from IF.

Myth #6 – Intermittent fasting is the sole reason for macronutrient deficiency.

Remember that if you follow your preferred intermittent fasting method the right way, you do not have to worry about experiencing nutrient deficiency. In fact, fasting is not the main reason for nutrient deficiency. Diet plans that are deficient in nutrients are actually the culprit. You will not suffer from nutrient deficiency if you actually stick to eating whole, balanced, and nutritious foods during your eating window.

You do not have to worry too much about your body not getting enough nutrients when you are fasting as there is no basis for such claim. In fact, fasting can cause your body to create nutrient efficiency. It increases the possibility of your body utilizing less nutrients, thereby retaining them so your body can efficiently use them in the future.

With that in mind, fasting can't be pointed as the culprit for nutrient deficiency but poor diet, chronic stress, unstable blood sugar levels, leaky gut syndrome, and low levels of stomach acid.

Myth #7 – Intermittent fasting can lead to overeating.

This is not true. What actually dictates your unhealthy eating behavior includes leptin and blood sugar. Having unstable blood sugar levels can cause food cravings, especially if your sugar crashes down. Being desensitized to leptin can also result in difficulties figuring out whether you have already consumed enough foods.

Leptin actually refers to a signaling hormone within your body, which plays a huge role in controlling your hunger. Certain factors, like chronic calorie restriction, poor quality of sleep, binge eating, and stress can lead to leptin resistance, causing you to be at a higher risk of overeating.

Instead of causing you to overeat, intermittent fasting can actually stabilize your blood sugar and improve your sensitivity to leptin. This can further improve your ability to control overeating or binge eating.

Myth #8 – You won't be able to exercise if you are fasting.

This is a misconception since it is actually safe for you to exercise even if you are on your fasting period. Working out will not result in muscle wasting or loss. In fact, fasted workouts can lead to the growth of your muscles provided you still consume adequate amounts of protein and calories every day.

In addition, working out while fasting can also produce other incredible benefits, including improved ketosis state, better fat burning ability, and increased growth hormone levels. Just make sure to stay hydrated if you intend to do some high-intensity exercises during your fasting state. In case you wish to gain muscles, then it would be helpful to take essential amino acid supplements.

Myth #9 – Intermittent fasting can lead to starving and irritability.

A lot of those who haven't tried intermittent fasting yet but want to do it for health reasons are often concerned about getting irritable if they experience extreme hunger. While this statement bears some weight, note that it is only true on a temporary basis.

You may experience irritability and hunger at first, especially if you are used to eating at least three meals spaced periodically every day. This may happen because you are still adjusting to your new eating routine/pattern.

You can't expect this to happen permanently, though. You can slowly make the adjustments by doing simple fasting routines or by doing it for one to two times every week at first. This will allow you to introduce the routine to your system. You can then slowly increase the number and duration of your fasting sessions as soon as you feel comfortable.

You do not have to rush things. Allow your body to adapt so you will not end up experiencing too much hunger and irritability. Once you are fully adjusted with this eating pattern, you can start enjoying its numerous benefits like better mental clarity and mood.

Myth #10 – Intermittent fasting does not work for those suffering from diabetes.

Another myth associated with fasting that you have to be aware of is that it is ineffective for diabetics. It is because most people are made to believe that they need to consume foods constantly as a means of maintaining their blood sugar level. The truth, however, is that IF works for those suffering from Type 2 diabetes, especially in improving weight loss results and stabilizing blood sugar.

There is even a possibility for prolonged fasting to restore their sensitivity to insulin. You may also combine IF with a ketogenic diet if you want to further improve its ability to restore your sensitivity to insulin. What is good about having improved insulin sensitivity is that your body will no longer need to produce too much insulin. This results in minimal inflammation, which is a big help for diabetics and those who are prone to developing kidney and heart diseases.

Type 1 diabetes sufferers who are incapable of producing insulin, however, should closely keep track of their blood sugar level before practicing intermittent fasting so they can do it correctly. They can still fast for around 12-16 hours every day but this will depend on the stability of their blood sugar level.

Chapter 8 – Unexpected Side Effects of Intermittent Fasting

While intermittent fasting is one of the most beneficial eating patterns that you can try at present, you still need to be extremely cautious before starting. Keep in mind that it is not risk-free. This makes it necessary to talk to your physician first and find out whether it is safe for you to follow this style of eating.

Also, find out if you have any health problem or complication that might cause the negative side effects, instead of rewarding benefits, of intermittent fasting to come out. It also helps to understand the most common side effects of intermittent fasting so you can study the whole approach carefully and find out how you can avoid them as much as possible.

- **Tiredness** – When doing IF, there is a high risk for you to experience tiredness and grogginess, especially if you are still a beginner. Take note that in this situation, your body will also most likely run on less energy than what it is used to. Fasting might also increase your stress level and disrupt your normal sleep patterns.

To avoid this specific side effect of intermittent fasting, it would be helpful for you to meditate or do other activities that will lower your stress levels. If you are working out on a regular basis, then consider scheduling it during your eating period. This is helpful in conserving your energy.

In addition, keep in mind that exercising while you are on the fasted state might lower your blood sugar level, which can trigger symptoms, like confusion and dizziness. It helps to be on the safe side by working out when you have already eaten.

- **Headaches** – You may be dealing with headaches because your body will tend to adjust to your new eating pattern. It could be caused by dehydration so it is advisable to drink plenty of water both during your eating window and fasting period. You may also experience headaches due to a sudden drop of your blood sugar level and the release of stress hormones during the fasting period.

The good news is that headaches usually happen only because your body is still on the adjustment stage. This means that this side effect is not permanent. Once you get used to it, you will no longer suffer from headaches.

- **Heartburn** – You may also experience heartburn due to fasting. In most cases, this problem will be resolved after around a couple of months. It is necessary to visit and consult your doctor in case your heartburn does not seem to resolve on its own even after your body has adjusted to the new eating pattern.

  Heartburn is often a result of your unfamiliarity to the fasting scenario, causing your body to release stomach acids automatically at certain times. While this can cause discomfort, this only happens at the beginning of your journey so there is no need for you to worry too much about it.

- **Brain fog** – This is also another common side effect of intermittent fasting, especially if your body is not yet used to the habit of not eating. This might cause your mind to try keeping up with the new routine, leading to confusion, forgetfulness, or brain fog. Once you familiarize yourself with how IF works, though, and your body has adjusted to the habit, you can expect better brain function from fasting.

- **Diarrhea** – Another unpleasant side effect of IF is diarrhea and it usually happens to those who are still beginners in fasting. There is even a higher risk for you to experience this problem if you enter the fasting period after consuming too much carbs. This problem may be associated to the significant drop in your insulin level, signaling your kidneys to get rid of excess water. This is the reason why you might experience unwanted and watery bowel movements.

You should also remember that your body tends to lose electrolytes via bowel movements and urination. If you experience watery stools or diarrhea, then one sign that you may experience at first is low level of sodium. With that in mind, it helps to drink broth or pickle juice during those days when you are dealing with this uncomfortable and unwanted IF side effect. It also helps to add around 1-2 pinches of salt in the water you drink.

- **Insomnia and anxiety** – Both these side effects may be caused by the production of adrenaline, a counter-regulatory hormone, when you begin to fast. In most cases, this effect is actually beneficial as it results in a high metabolic rate and energy level. The problem is that the energy you get from it might be too high even during those specific times when you are supposed to be sleeping.

This can also make you feel jittery and anxious. It could be because of consuming too much coffee especially during the beginning of your fasting journey. Your anxiety also tends to worsen if you constantly worry about the effects of fasting to your health. You can resolve these side effects by sticking to proper bedtime routines, such as turning off your gadgets and electronics ninety minutes prior to your bedtime. You can also relax with the help of Epsom salt baths.

- **Bad breath** – Another unpleasant and unexpected side effect of intermittent fasting is bad breath. This often happens if you already start losing weight due to fasting. This side effect is also referred to as the keto breath characterized by your tongue becoming white and a taste of acetone in your mouth. It is mainly because acetone is known as the by-product of metabolizing fatty acid.

A lot of those who tried fasting and experienced the keto breath tend to freak out upon noticing their white tongues. They even wrongly assume that it is a result of nutrient deficiency. If this happens to you then avoid freaking out. This is actually your body's normal reaction to the fat-burning process.

As weight loss starts slowing down, you will notice a great improvement in your breath. You will also notice your tongue going back to its normal pink color. If you really feel uncomfortable with this side effect then there are some things that you can do to manage it. One is to brush your teeth as frequently as possible all throughout the day. Drinking more water and using a tongue scraper can also help.

Intermittent fasting provides numerous benefits to those who are obese, overweight, and have average weight. However, it is not appropriate for everyone, including pregnant and breastfeeding women and those who are dealing with eating disorders and certain health issues.

This is the main reason why you have to study the effects of fasting to you as soon as you begin doing it. Listen to your own body. If you notice some unwanted side effects, find out if it is because your body is just adjusting to the routine or due to more serious issues. If you are extremely worried about the negative side effects, do not hesitate to consult your doctor to ensure your safety.

Chapter 9 – Intermittent Fasting Mistakes that You Should Avoid Committing

Sticking to an intermittent fasting approach will let you experience tremendous benefits, among which are better digestion, significant weight loss, minimal sugar cravings, better sleep, and improved mental clarity. However, your journey towards attaining your desired results will most likely be accompanied with some errors.

While you can't perfect intermittent fasting for the entire period you are planning to do it, take note that there are some mistakes committed by other practitioners of this eating pattern that you can simply avoid.

Mistake #1 – Changing your eating habits drastically

If you are one of those whose normal eating habits include eating every three to four hours or so then shrinking the time you need to eat within just an 8-hour period all of a sudden can lead to certain issues, like extreme hunger and frustration. A lot of people make the mistake of adding drastic changes into their lifestyle and eating patterns all of a sudden by trying to stick to a long fasting period.

This can lead to quitting after just a short period of fasting because they experienced difficulties in adjusting from their previous eating behaviors and habits. You should avoid this mistake as much as possible if you want to succeed in IF. Always remember that you might need around 10-14 days to finally adjust and prevent yourself from feeling extreme hunger during your fasting period. Avoid making the change in your eating habits all of a sudden.

What you have to do, instead, is to stretch the amount of time in between your meals in a gradual manner (for instance, until you reach an eating window of 12 hours). You should then move into an eating window of 10 hours. After that, reduce that window even further but only by small increments. Do this until you reached your target eating window.

Mistake #2 – Consuming the wrong liquids

Some people drink tea, black coffee, or water so they can go through their fasting period with the least amount of discomfort. The problem is that if you can't tolerate black coffee then you may be tempted to add some sugar or milk without thinking about whether or not this will break your fast. Prior to adding anything to your drink, find out if it will affect your desired results first. If possible, do not let coconut oil and butter get near your coffee.

You should also stay away from liquids filled with protein, like bone broth. It is because these liquids have the ability to stop autophagy, which refers to a cellular process capable of breaking down and recycling damaged molecules. This is something that you may want to achieve when you are on your fasting period.

It is also advisable to stay away from diet sodas. You need to avoid anything, which is sweetened heavily, even those advertised as free of calories. Remember that even zero-calorie sweeteners can negatively affect your insulin level, which might also stimulate your appetite and cause cravings.

To prevent taking in wrong liquids, keep track of your hydration and the specific drinks you take in. This is a huge help in making yourself accountable and motivating yourself to stick to black coffee, plain tea, and water during the fasting period. Once you get used to drinking the right liquids, make sure that you do not forget to hydrate yourself, especially during the fasted state.

Note that while the IF regiment refrains you from eating foods during your fasting period, it is necessary for water or other healthy liquids to be close to you. It is mainly because this eating pattern might cause you to miss out on the kind of hydration often provided by healthy fruits and vegetables.

You do not want to suffer from dehydration as it has several side effects, like muscle cramps, hunger pangs, and headaches. With that in mind, ensure that you sip enough water and other allowed liquids all throughout the day regardless if you are in your eating or fasting window.

Mistake #3 – Leading a sedentary lifestyle

Working out when you are sticking to the intermittent fasting approach might seem like a new endeavor for you, especially if you are used to eating a pre-workout snack. However, this should not be a reason why you should lead a sedentary lifestyle during your fasted state. Note that even if you are fasting, you can't still lose weight if you do not pair it with proper exercise.

The good news is that your body actually stores plenty of energy in your body fat. This is what your body will use in case there is no food. With that in mind, it is possible for you to retain your usual exercise routines even when you have changed your eating pattern. If the entire experience is really new then you may want to try out low-impact exercises, like walking.

In case you decide to fast overnight and work out during the morning then it is advisable to consume a meal rich in protein after it. It is helpful in increasing your body's muscle-building rate. One thing to remember before pairing IF with your regular workout, though, is that just like other exercise or diet plans, you have to consult your doctor first. However, in general, pairing your regular exercises with IF is safe.

Mistake #4 – Sticking to the wrong intermittent fasting plan or approach.

Note that for IF to produce favorable results, you need to pick the right plan – one that perfectly fits your lifestyle, current condition, and personality. Avoid making yourself miserable by trying to stick to a pattern, which is not compatible with your own lifestyle. If you know that you are a night owl, for instance, then avoid starting your fasting sessions every 6 pm.

In case you are someone who goes to the gym every day and do not want to sacrifice your daily workout then avoid picking an IF plan/method, which has severe calorie restrictions for several days every week. Consider your lifestyle and personality and find out which among the IF methods will work for you. By choosing the most suitable fasting method, it will be easier for you to stick to the new habit.

Mistake #5 – Beating yourself up in case you eat beyond your eating window

Do not feel too guilty if you slip up from the pattern sometimes. Avoid beating yourself up when you grab a food even if you are no longer in your eating window. Note that you need to listen to the cues sent by your body. If you feel real hunger then there is no reason to deprive yourself of what you need.

Remember that addressing your hunger is actually okay when doing intermittent fasting. Just make sure that you do not do it all the time. Also, one thing that you have to remind yourself on a constant basis is that if you deny your body's hunger cues then your relationship with food will become unhealthy.

Do not be too hard on yourself and allow it to break from the fast in case you truly feel hungry during your supposed-to-be fasting state. Keep in mind that the idea behind intermittent fasting is not to starve yourself. With that in mind, it is crucial to still provide yourself with the right nourishment, especially if you are starting to experience negative symptoms.

Mistake #6 – Restricting calories too much when the eating window comes

One problem experienced by those who just started following intermittent fasting is that the whole eating pattern causes them to continue restricting their calories even after breaking their fast. You do not have to be too strict and rigid by excessively restricting your calorie intake. Note that intermittent fasting also requires you to hear what your body is telling you. Listen to it and eat until you experience fullness.

The good news is that the human body is actually an incredible machine but you also have to let it to do its job correctly. In that case, you can expect it to release hormones that will let you know whether you are already full. You just have to watch out for the 1 it releases that signify fullness.

Avoid restricting your calorie intake too much during the time when you are supposed to eat. It is because doing so might only lead to under-eating, causing several unwanted body changes and long-term consequences.

Mistake #7 – Pushing yourself too hard

This is a mistake often committed by those who wish to try extending their fast for as long as possible even if it means forcing themselves. Some even go to the extent of fasting for more than 48 hours even if they already experience too much discomfort. You should determine whether the extended/prolonged fast works for you before trying it out first.

Keep in mind that you can't expect the process of extending your fast to supercharge IF and produce more incredible benefits. If you force yourself to fast for an extremely long period even to the point of extreme discomfort then consider seeking the help of a counselor whose specialty is on eating disorders. The foods you regularly eat should not cause regret and remorse, so seeking the help of a professional can be beneficial.

Also, take note that your poor relationship with food can produce even bigger problems in the future. This is why talking to a counselor is really advisable so you can figure out whether you already have an eating disorder or if your relationship with food is still healthy.

Mistake #8 – Obsessing over eating windows and schedules

One great benefit of intermittent fasting is that it teaches you to be fully in tune with your own body signals. It allows you to understand real hunger, which is something that happens every 16 to 24 hours instead of the every 4 hours that a lot of people believe. With that in mind, you do not have to obsess too much over your eating windows and schedules.

You have to make sure that your body dictates the perfect time for you to eat, instead of the clock. Focusing on time periods too much might cause you to count the hours left until your next meal. This will prevent you from learning and fully understanding the signals sent to you by your own body.

For instance, if you decide to skip breakfast then you are basically extending your fasting overnight to around 16 hours. Your focus should not be on the schedule or the time period. This means that in case you decide to skip breakfast, then you also have the option of breaking the fast once you feel hungry, although it is advisable to do this only occasionally.

Mistake #9 – Trying to do numerous things at once

You may be forcing yourself to do a lot of things while trying to practice the intermittent fasting approach. Some of the things you might do are over-training, dry fasting, and under-eating. Also, remember that if you are someone with poor eating habits and who lacks workout in the past and want to try intermittent fasting for better health then avoid biting more than what you can actually chew. This is important, especially if you are still a beginner.

Allow yourself to ease gradually into training and fasting. Also, avoid training 5 times weekly, fasting daily, and extremely restricting your calorie intake after fasting.

It is because this might only trigger serious consequences in the future. One more thing to remind yourself is that your body survives with a bit of physical stress from time to time. However, you should try avoiding too much stress as this might produce more chronic issues.

Mistake #10 – Choosing the wrong foods

A lot of intermittent fasting followers also make the mistake of choosing the wrong foods. In fact, many of those who tried it think that it is a magic pill capable of solving their weight and health problems. While it is true that IF is an effective tool for those who want to have full control over their health and weight, it is still possible to cancel out its benefits if you eat the wrong foods, specifically processed and sugary ones, during your eating window.

Keep in mind that since you are fasting, it is more essential to give your body the right nourishment through whole and nutrient-dense foods. Being in the fasted state also encourages your body to break down any damaged parts then use these to produce energy. This is helpful in healing and cleansing your body. This also results to in body becoming more and more sensitive to all the foods you take in. Such sensitivity is beneficial if you take in foods rich in nutrients.

However, it will not do you any good if the foods you consume do not nourish your body. If that is the case, you will experience extreme hunger most of the time since your body will start to crave for nutrients. With that in mind, focus on consuming highly nutritious foods when it is already time to eat. Do not just focus on cutting calories. Your goal is to ensure that your body still receives sufficient amount of nutritious foods to ensure that your organs and your brain will continue to function well.

To avoid this mistake, read the next chapter of this book to figure out some of the healthiest foods that you can take during your eating window.

Chapter 10 – The Best Foods to Eat During the Eating Window

Intermittent fasting is one of the key solutions for your body to clean out and repair any cellular junk that you have accumulated for several years. This results in the improved function of your body organs and systems. However, you can't expect this eating pattern to perform such an important role successfully if you do not support it with adequate amounts of nutritious foods. The right foods are essential in the process of replenishing and rebuilding your body.

You have to pick whole and good foods with high nutrient density. Eventually, your body will master the art of signaling when it already had enough foods. In return, you will also master the art of listening to your body cues. This will allow you to eat less than what you normally consume before without being too restrictive.

Another thing that you have to remember about intermittent fasting is that it will not work if you follow an extremely restrictive diet. It is because this might cause you to be extremely starved physically and emotionally. This might result in you overeating due to deprivation, so avoid making yourself feel too hungry unnecessarily for a long period.

Just make sure to avoid sticking to processed and unhealthy foods. You still need a well-balanced diet rich in whole and nutritious foods for intermittent fasting to help you in reaching your weight loss and health goals.

So what are the best foods to eat during your eating window? Here are some of the most nutritious ones:

- **Whole Grains** – Carbs are actually vital for your health. In fact, you can't consider them as your mortal enemy when trying to lose weight. Note that since you are practicing intermittent fasting, a huge chunk of your daily routine will be spent on the fasted state.

- With that in mind, you need to look for a strategic solution to obtain enough calories without overeating. Yes, you will need to minimize processed foods but you can also include some from time to time, like whole grain breads, crackers, and bagels.

It is because your body can quickly digest these foods, giving you a good supply of fuel in an instant. They also serve as excellent sources of energy if you are training or exercising regularly while doing the fast. What is good about whole grains is that they also have high amounts of protein and fiber. This means that you do not have to eat too much of it to keep yourself full.

It is also advisable to eat whole grains instead of the refined ones as the former can improve your metabolism. Among the healthiest whole grains that you can include in your diet to further improve the results of IF are amaranth, sorghum, millet, spelt, and bulgur.

- **Lentil** – This is a highly nutritious food, which is rich in fiber. In fact, one-half cup of it can already provide up to 32% of the total amount of fiber you need every day. Aside from fiber, lentil is also rich in iron, which is good if you are an active female who is also trying to stick to intermittent fasting.

- **Potatoes** – Just like bread, potatoes can also be digested by your body with the least amount of effort. Pairing it with a good source of protein can turn it into a great post-workout snack designed to refuel your hungry and tired muscles.

  Another advantage of including potatoes in your regular diet if you are following the intermittent fasting approach is that they are effective in forming a resistant starch, which can fuel the good bacteria present in your gut.

- **Nuts** – While the calorie content of nuts is higher compared to other snacks, they are still good for your body because they have an important component not present in the majority of junk foods – that is good fat.

In fact, you can take advantage of the polyunsaturated fat present in walnut to change the physiological markers linked to both satiety and hunger, making this snack really beneficial for intermittent fasters.

- **Eggs** – Even one piece of large egg already contains up to 6 grams of protein, which is helpful in making yourself feel full as well as in the muscle-building process. Another advantage of eggs is that they are easy and quick to prepare. They are ready within just a few minutes. Hard-boiled eggs are also both filling and nutritious, making them perfect additions to your eating window.

- **Berries** – Different kinds of berries can also help fill you up while providing your body with essential nutrients. Strawberries, for instance, are excellent sources of Vitamin C, which can boost your immunity. You can also eat blueberries that have high flavonoid content.

There are also fiber-rich raspberries that are great additions to your diet. Note that each cup of raspberries already contains 8 grams of fiber, keeping you full and regular even during your shortened eating window.

- **Fish** – Intermittent fasting can produce even better results for you if you include fish in your eating schedule. Aside from having high protein and healthy fat content, different kinds of fish are also rich in Vitamin D.

It provides sufficient amount of nutrients, which is great if your food intake will be limited only to your eating window. What's good about fish is that it is also considered as a brain food, which is great during the times when you are restricting your calorie intake that might affect your cognition.

- **Cruciferous Vegetables** – These include cauliflower, Brussels sprouts, and broccoli – all of which have high fiber content. Note that erratic eating caused by adapting the intermittent fasting approach to weight loss requires you to consume more fiber-rich foods to avoid constipation and keep you regular. What is great about fiber is that it also leads to fullness, which is beneficial especially if you are planning to go through the day with most hours spent on fasting.

- **Legumes and beans** – Adapting the IF lifestyle might prompt you to fall in love with legumes and beans that are rich in low-calorie carbs that can supply you with enough energy for your daily activities. This makes them vital additions to your eating plan. Also, foods that belong to the legume and bean family including black beans, lentils, peas, and chickpeas can significantly reduce your body weight even if you do not restrict your calorie intake.

Following the intermittent fasting lifestyle can indeed give you desirable results but you have to make sure that you are also helping yourself by eating the right foods. Make sure that when you break the fast, your focus is on foods rich in essential vitamins and protein.

These nutrients are necessary in boosting your immunity. It also helps to add fiber-rich foods into your eating plan to ensure that your digestive system continues to work properly. Go for olive oil, tomatoes, oily fish, and nuts.

You should also know what foods to stay away from. Avoid refined carbs, including chips, cakes, biscuits, and sugar as your body might convert these foods to fat quickly. If you wish to eat foods with a lower calorie content than usual then ensure that the calories are as nutritious and as good for your body as possible.

Note that just because you need to eat calories does not mean that you should get these calories from low-quality and unhealthy sources.

Chapter 11 – Frequently Asked Questions about Intermittent Fasting

As a bonus chapter, spend time checking out the most frequently asked questions about intermittent fasting so you will get to know more about this highly beneficial eating pattern and lifestyle.

Who can benefit from intermittent fasting?

Taking into consideration the benefits and side effects of intermittent fasting, this lifestyle is suitable for those who enjoy different kinds of food and struggle sticking to diet plans that are too restrictive on certain macronutrients and food groups. It is because the main focus of IF is not the quantity and quality of food you eat but the timeframe.

This means that if there are certain foods you want to eat, like pasta or chocolate, then you can just patiently wait for your eating window so you can enjoy them. Just do not forget to enjoy them in moderation and still include healthy and nutritious foods into your eating plan. It also works great for those suffering from digestive issues at night.

It is because bumping up their last daily meal before bedtime aids in preventing acid reflux, heartburn, and other digestive issues. What is even better about IF is that it has different versions with varying levels of difficulty, which does not necessarily make it a one-size-fits-all solution. This means anyone can decide and determine what IF method can benefit them the most.

Who should not try intermittent fasting?

IF is not suitable for pregnant and breastfeeding women who need nutrients to support their growing babies. Also, take note that while fasting is beneficial in controlling blood sugar, diabetics who are dependent to insulin still need to avoid radical fasting methods.

Note that these patients need to enjoy healthy and regular meals as a means of preventing sudden spikes and dips in their blood sugar level that might be damaging to them if uncontrolled. Intermittent fasting is not also suitable for professional and amateur athletes who are dependent on perfectly timed fuel prior to and after each activity so they can improve their athletic performance and ability to recover fast.

Can I work out even on an empty stomach?

This question is actually tough because the answer is dependent on one's goal. One thing to take note of, though, is that if you have not consumed food for quite a while then it is greatly possible for your glycogen or energy stores to be depleted.

Also, the ketosis mechanism designed to burn fat to convert it into fuel would have barely started. That said, it is possible that you will not have the required energy to work out, especially if you intend to stick to a high-intensity routine.

In case your goal is to retain your muscle mass during intermittent fasting then it is not advisable to work out on an empty stomach. Keep in mind that maintaining muscle mass often requires you to do some heavy lifting activities. You can't do that if you feel too weak because you are still on the fasting period. This is the main reason why it is not advisable to strength-train when you have an empty stomach.

If your main goal is to lose excess fats then performing medium-intensity cardio workouts during your fasting period can produce more desirable results. It is because this helps in kick-starting your ketosis mechanism, leading to weight loss. With these different answers, remember that whether or not you should work out on an empty stomach will always depend on your ultimate fitness goals.

Will my body burn muscles if I fast?

No, your body will not burn muscles when you fast. Remember that the idea that your body will use muscle rather than the fat stored within for energy is a misconception. What your body is looking for is actually efficiency. It will be inefficient if your body will burn lean muscles or body mass instead of stored energy.

You can only expect your body to burn lean body mass in case it can't detect any stored energy, like when you are starving yourself and this is not what happens when you are fasting since it does not actually involve complete starvation.

Also, remember that most people have above normal body mass index, which means that there is no need to worry about your body burning muscles in order to produce fuel.

How can intermittent fasting help in weight loss?

One reason why many try to practice intermittent fasting is to lose weight and you can expect it to work wonders in that area. It is possible for fasting to aid in weight loss because it also results in a drop of your insulin level. Insulin refers to a storage hormone, which works by taking out sugar from your blood, allowing it to work in reducing your blood sugar.

It then uses that sugar in using or storing energy. You can also expect insulin to move energy, which already appears as glucose, into your muscle cells that when full will further move the energy into your liver. This will then result to stored fats.

All the foods you eat can actually increase the level of your insulin. If you are fasting then it will subsequently reduce your insulin level. Without insulin in your system, you will not be able to store energy. It will cause your body to tap into your stored energy which is now in the form of fat, to produce fuel, thereby resulting in weight loss.

Is it okay to add some milk or cream to my coffee when fasting?

Yes. You do not have to be too rigid on what you drink during your fasting period. Adding milk or cream, therefore, will not cause a lot of harm to your results. Also, remember that fasting tends to work due to its ability to maintain the low levels of your insulin, allowing it to continue stimulating the fat burning process.

How can I maintain the results I got so far with intermittent fasting?

If you have already reached your weight loss goal through intermittent fasting then your next step is to be on a maintenance mode. In this case, you are allowed to cycle your carbs and calories every day depending on the level of your hunger and your activity. Know exactly what your maintenance level calories should be on a daily basis. Make sure to base it on your activity level, gender, age, height, and new weight.

Can I adapt intermittent fasting on a long-term basis?

Of course. In fact, IF can be considered as a long-term solution to weight loss. Through intermittent fasting, you no longer have to follow ineffective diet plans anymore. Many even view IF as the easiest way for you to live and stay lean. Note that in most cases, short-lived diet plans fail.

It is even possible that your short-lived attempts to lose weight are the specific reasons why you continue gaining weight. If you do not follow the diet plan forever then it will also fail you. Intermittent fasting, on the other hand, can't be considered as a diet plan. It is an eating pattern and lifestyle, which tells you about the specific times when you can and can't eat.

With that in mind, it is much easier to stick to it for a longer period. It can shed your unwanted fats while ensuring that you stay lean for a long time. What is even better about it is that it requires minimal effort, especially once you become used to it, so maintaining it as a long-term solution is possible.

Conclusion

Intermittent fasting continues to receive global exposure nowadays considering its numerous incredible benefits. It is true that this popular eating pattern is beneficial and favorable for your health, wellbeing and weight, but you also have to make sure that you do it properly. Also, remember that just like other diet plans, this eating pattern can't provide you with your desired results overnight. You need to have patience and discipline to be able to reap its benefits.

For instance, if you feel a strong urge to eat, find out first if it is real hunger or just plain craving. If you are just craving for something, then fill yourself with a low-calorie snack or water. You can also successfully go through the fasting state by keeping yourself busy. This is helpful in distracting yourself from eating. It also helps to start slow and allow your body to adjust to the routine at its own pace.

You have to learn the ins and outs of intermittent fasting before trying it out so you can reap its full benefits in a sustainable and safe manner. It is effective not only in losing weight but also in reducing oxidative stress associated with cancer and aging. It even helps you live longer. This approach is safe to practice for the majority of overweight people. However, make sure to consult your doctor first, especially if you have an illness before planning to practice this approach.